Dirty Talk

The Definitive Instruction Manual On Enhancing
Intimacy Through Written Communication

*(Inspiring Declarations That Can Evoke Passion And
Intensify Arousal In Her Right Away)*

I0082886

Jaime Cotton

TABLEO OF CONTENT

Illustrative Instances Of Being In Each Other's Company In A Public Setting

One of my preferred methods of arousing sexual tension involves discreetly murmuring phrases into my partner's ear during public or social gatherings. These are circumstances in which immediate physical intimacy is not possible. By creating distance between the desire for sex and the actual event of sex you are able to create massive amounts of tension.

Below are some appropriate responses to employ when engaging with your partner in public scenarios that may preclude immediate physical affection. Instances where this might occur include attending a social gathering or a professional function. This intensifies the sexual tension due to its highly forbidden nature. Attempt to discreetly communicate the following phrases directly into your male companion's ear. Articulating these words audibly in the presence of individuals nearby can amplify their erotic impact. Please exercise caution to avoid detection.

Examples In Public

Please refrain from directing your gaze towards me in such a manner. You're turning me on.

Fortunately, your inability to perceive my current thoughts is quite advantageous. There are numerous actions I deeply desire to undertake towards you.

Unfortunately, due to our current surroundings, I find it regrettable that there are numerous desires I hold towards you, and I am uncertain of my ability to exhibit further patience.

I specifically chose to don this dress/skirt/jeans/outfit solely with the intention of pleasing you.

I have an unexpected revelation in store for you once we arrive home later.

I am not currently donning any undergarments. I would be delighted to demonstrate, do you happen to be aware of a suitable venue?

If there were an occasion on which you were to return home one evening and discover me in a vulnerable state, specifically, positioned in an exposed manner upon the bed, eagerly anticipating your intimate engagement, what course of action would you choose to undertake?

Are there any particular preferences or desires that you would be interested in exploring this evening? The atmosphere of this party/event is arousing, making me yearn to engage in intimate activities with you.

It proves challenging to engage in social interactions at this gathering, as my primary inclination is to discreetly accompany you to a more private setting for intimate connection.

I am intrigued, what is the most risqué activity you have ever contemplated engaging in with me? If we weren't at this party/event I might just let you.

May I inquire about the anticipated end time of this party/event, as I find myself growing impatient and my thoughts consumed by the desire for our intimate encounter?

Utilize Literature Suitable For The Respective Age Group

In recent years, there has been a proliferation of sex education books accessible on the internet.

It can be challenging to broach the topic of sexuality with one's children. Nonetheless, owing to the accessibility of literature on sexual education tailored to different age groups, discussing the subject of sexuality with your child can be approached effortlessly.

As your child matures, it is only natural for them to express curiosity regarding matters concerning sex, and it is essential that they receive accurate and informative answers.

Based on research, books that are suitable for a child's age can be employed as a starting point for initiating discussions about topics related to human sexuality with your child.

Books can serve as a contingency option in the event that a conversation completely disintegrates.

The Advantages of Engaging with Literature Tailored to One's Age Group

If you are genuinely interested in engaging in a conversation with your child regarding human reproduction and sexuality, it is advisable to familiarize yourself with literature specifically tailored to facilitate these discussions with age-appropriate content. If you are a parent seeking age-appropriate books for your child, rest assured that there is a substantial range of options available this year, alleviating any concerns you may have.

With the aid of these books, your adolescent will acquire enhanced understanding of the intricacies pertaining to human sexuality and its practical implications.

A wide range of age-appropriate sex novels cater to diverse age groups, facilitating an effortless selection of the finest literary works suitable for your child's age.

By providing your child with these age-appropriate educational materials on sexuality, you can rest assured that they will gain valuable knowledge and have their inquiries addressed with accuracy and authenticity.

There exist numerous strategies to initiate a conversation regarding human sexuality with your child, and the aid of these literary works shall greatly facilitate your ability to articulate and steer them through this subject matter with efficiency and efficacy.

The prevailing viewpoint among adolescents is that their parents exert the greatest influence over them, particularly with regard to matters concerning sexuality. Adolescents who engage in favorably interactive experiences with their parents and engage in age-appropriate literary pursuits display an increased propensity to delay sexual initiation, employ contraceptive measures such as condoms, and maintain fewer sexual partners.

As a parent, it is incumbent upon you to fulfill your responsibility by providing guidance and addressing your child's sexual development and sexual matters. Upon hearing the term "sexuality," what is the initial thought that comes to your mind?

Sexuality encompasses a comprehensive exploration of the mechanics of the female and male anatomy, the intricacies of various types of relationships, processes of reproduction, stages of human development, preventative measures against sexually transmitted infections and unwanted pregnancy, as well as the nuances surrounding sexual conduct.

Undoubtedly, broaching the subjects of avian and insect reproduction with one's child can pose challenges; however, by utilizing literature that is suitable for their age, it is possible to effectively elucidate the fundamental principles of human sexual behavior and identity.

Certain parents have the intention of imparting comprehensive knowledge about human sexuality to their children in a singular, extended conversation, which often involves planning and engaging in discussions on this topic over the course of several months. Conversely, parents may experience frustration if the dialogue deviates from the anticipated course. Engaging in an ongoing conversation with your child regarding matters of sexuality and sex is imperative, as it should be a discourse that endures throughout their lifetime.

In order to mitigate ambiguity and inquisitiveness, it is imperative to engage in a prompt conversation with your child. When your child's inquisitiveness emerges, this presents a prime occasion to engage in a dialogue with them. You will observe a profound cultivation of trust and mutual respect between you and your child as a result of this conversation, which will

undoubtedly   bring   you   great
satisfaction.

If you happen to have young offspring, it is advisable to motivate them to engage with literature precisely tailored to their age group, as this will facilitate their acquisition of anatomical terminology pertaining to the different parts of their physique.   When   engaging   in conversations about sexuality with your child, it is essential to ensure that the content remains suitable for their age and development level. They will acquire enhanced capacity to address the subject matter with greater ease and grasp the complexities   pertaining   to   sex   and sexuality as an outcome.

The Guidelines for Engaging in Erotic Conversation

Now   that   you   have   acquired   an understanding of what actions to avoid, it will become more manageable to direct your attention towards the positive measures you can take to enhance the intimacy within the confines of the bedroom.

Prepare Yourself

The mere act of exploring techniques to enhance sexual experiences through the acquisition of knowledge on erotic language situates you in a position of advantage compared to a multitude of individuals. Nonetheless, it should be acknowledged that you still have ample room for growth and further acquisition of knowledge. Please ensure that you are adequately prepared. It is advisable to give prior thought to the points you would like to articulate. Whether you employ your creative faculties or utilize the expressions provided within this literary work, locate a point of origination in which you feel at ease. Select phrases that exhibit smoothness when articulated and subsequently commit them to memory.

Engaging in this exercise will result in a decreased tendency to experience a loss for words when expressing sexual desires or responding to a partner's request for erotic communication. Moreover, this approach will assist you in preventing the utterance of phrases that appear clumsy, comedic, or foolish, especially when your intention is to exude sensuality.

Check Your Tone

Develop your speaking voice. This is an activity that can be honed and refined through consistent practice and cultivation. Locate a tranquil and secluded space in which you may engage in the cultivation of an agreeable vocal quality. Refrain from raising your voice excessively, yet avoid speaking too softly. Please make an effort to articulate clearly and speak at a moderate pace.

If you are in a relationship with a partner who displays submissiveness during intimate moments, it is recommended to refine your communication skills by adopting a authoritative vocal demeanor. It is more challenging than one might anticipate.

Ensure that you maintain proper control over your non-verbal cues as well. Please maintain proper posture by aligning your shoulders, ensuring a stable position for your hands, and regulating your breathing in a composed manner.

In the event that your partner exhibits a dominant nature, it is advisable to employ a reserved yet sufficiently audible vocal expression. This section pertains to discerning your partner's preferences and integrating them with your own sensual inclinations.

Sustain visual engagement, but avoid prolonged fixations.

Maintaining proper eye contact is imperative; however, it is crucial to avoid the misconception of prolonged staring. You ought to make an effort to maintain eye contact intermittently. This is particularly crucial in the event that you offer a compliment to someone. Eye contact adds credibility. Additionally, employing direct eye contact with your partner as you communicate your desires can greatly intensify the impact and effectivenesss of your words. Exercising restraint is crucial. Ponder your opportunities judiciously.

Know Your Boundaries

Should you possess a certain level of familiarity with your significant other, you may already possess knowledge regarding permissible topics or subjects that ought to be avoided in conversation. If they possess an aversion towards profanities, they may not find it agreeable when you engage in the use of expletives. An effective approach to determining their linguistic preferences is by observing the manner in which they discuss their own physical being. In the event that they refer to their breasts exclusively as "breasts," it is advised to employ that specific terminology. When individuals demonstrate a willingness to employ more explicit language, only then may you utilize such terminology.

This is just a general guide though. There are individuals who hold conservative views but would exhibit great enthusiasm upon hearing explicit expressions. This is something you'll understand better in time though, so keep working on it with your partner.

Please ensure effective communication with your partner and acquaint yourself with their personal preferences. Initiating that conversation may appear somewhat daunting, however, by courteously inquiring about their preferences and aversions, it will mark the commencement of a necessary discussion.

Know Your Partner

This is closely correlated with understanding and respecting personal limits, thus emphasizing its criticality warrants our undivided attention. Prior to engaging in explicit conversation, it is advisable to possess a fundamental understanding of your partner's preferences and desires regarding intimate communication during sexual encounters. Do they have an affinity for intimate encounters characterized by tenderness? Rough? Perhaps they are eager to explore numerous unconventional positions. Do they utilize sexual aids? What are their sentiments regarding bondage and S&M practices? Being unaware of their preferences necessitates a considerable amount of conjecture, thus entailing potential risks. This presents an opportune moment to acquaint oneself with one's partner in such a manner. Acquire knowledge about their preferences and remember to consider them when contemplating suggestive phrases to share with them during intimate moments.

If you happen to be disinclined, there is no need for you to make a direct inquiry of them. One can acquire knowledge of these preferences by attentively observing one's partner and engaging in novel experiences together. However, the most convenient and direct approach would be to inquire with them. If you experience significant discomfort or encounter difficulty broaching the subject, one potential approach would be to engage in joint viewing of erotic or pornographic films. Engage in a discourse about the content you have viewed and deliberate upon pleasurable activities you wish to partake in. Additionally, make a point of observing the factors that caused your displeasure. Once both individuals are at ease discussing matters pertaining to sexuality, it will considerably facilitate the process of establishing a deeper understanding of one another.

Maintain concise and succinct communication (or, alternatively, concise and direct communication).

Monologues are certainly regarded with disapproval. Avoid the inclination to deliver a scholarly discourse if your aim is to engage in seductive conversation and ignite passion in your partner. Effective erotic communication hinges on the prowess of one's creative faculties, with verbal expression serving as a mere catalyst for the ensuing gratification of physical senses. Continuing to discuss it at length will create an uncomfortable and disruptive atmosphere.

Be Natural

Please only articulate sentiments with which you feel at ease. It will be quite evident if you are compelled to articulate sentiments with which you do not concur, or when you lack assurance. Do not attempt to assume an identity that is not authentic to your true self, however, this should not discourage you from embracing and pursuing calculated ventures. Engage in diligent practice and strive for excellence. If certain circumstances cause you to experience blushing, there is no cause for concern. It is not necessary for you to verbalize it. Ensure that you maintain your true identity.

Change Your Expressions

It is customary to experience a sense of unease or self-consciousness when engaging in explicit conversation for the first time. Nevertheless, be sure to maintain a composed yet alluring countenance during the act. If one is experiencing a substantial amount of enjoyment, it is permissible to engage in smiling. Additionally, coy smiles can be effective when uttering suggestive remarks. It is advisable to refrain from wearing an overly lighthearted expression, as it may cause confusion and potentially even offend your partner.

Share Your Fantasies

Communicating your most provocative fantasies to your significant other serves as an exceptional method of engaging in explicit discussion that simultaneously ignites their imagination. Explore the possibility of both of you satisfying those desires. This arrangement is most suitable when both parties have established a high level of mutual comfort, as it facilitates genuine self-expression. Do not hesitate to express your long-desired aspirations to them. Observe how it stimulates their excitement.

The disadvantage is that one must exercise a certain degree of caution. Certain fantasies may not be well received by your romantic partner.

Ensure that you have the ability to articulate your most intimate and private desires without apprehension of being subjected to scrutiny.

Start Soft

This advice is highly beneficial for individuals who are new to the subject/area/activity. Prior to engaging in overtly explicit language, you may consider gradually introducing auditory expressions such as groans, sighs, moans, and other vocalizations that effectively convey the intensity of the pleasure you are currently experiencing. At this juncture, it is imperative that you feel at ease with your vocal prowess. If your partner also emits vocalizations, it is an indication of your achievement.

Discover the factors that incite excitement and arousal within you and your significant other.

Discovering what causes you to experience a sense of uncleanliness is a captivating journey. In order to discover your authentic 'voice', it is essential to engage in introspection. The subsequent inquiries will aid in your discovery. If you are able to facilitate your partner's participation in answering these questions, it would be highly beneficial given that both of you will gain precise insight into each other's desires.

It would be advisable to document your responses. Recording the aforementioned ideas in writing, as opposed to mere contemplation, will enhance your level of consciousness.

When one is sexually aroused and experiences feelings of impurity...

What is the term or designation you use when addressing or alluding to your significant other?

What are the terms used to refer to your erogenous zones?

What term do you utilize to designate the erogenous areas of your significant other?

Does the manner in which you address yourself undergo any alterations? May I inquire if there is an alternative appellation that you prefer?

At what time would you prefer to engage in explicit communication? Do you derive pleasure from auditory stimuli during the sexual experience? Do you wish to receive this information within the context of foreplay? Most times? Occasionally? Rarely?

What emotions do you experience when engaging in provocative speech? Are you submissive? Neutral? Dominant? Slight shades of each?

At what point would you be interested in engaging in explicit discourse with your romantic partner? Immediately? Soon? When you become more acquainted with them? Never?

Do you find comfort in being reduced to an object of admiration? In what way?

Would you rather be addressed using offensive language? If yes, which terms?

Do you have a propensity for using profane language?

Do you find it agreeable when your significant other uses profanity?

Do you have any inclination to dehumanize or reduce the value of your partner during intimate conversation? In what way?

Although these inquiries may appear abundant, acquiring knowledge of the corresponding responses will undeniably have a beneficial impact on your sexual well-being. The initial phase in attaining one's preferences is to ascertain one's preferences. The aforementioned applies to your significant other as well.

How to Induce Attraction in a Woman Through Non-Physical Means

Speak Like A Detective.

One of the initial observations that must be made is that an individual's vocal expression serves as a means through which their social positioning is communicated to others. It is of utmost significance to enhance the efficacy of your vocal expression in order to captivate the attention of a woman without any physical contact.

Please refrain from elevating your voice at the conclusion of your sentences during conversation. Lower your vocal tone towards the end of each sentence. When one concludes sentences seamlessly, it inherently conveys a sense of authority and effectively influences the mental state of the listener through the display of dominance. This is the undisclosed knowledge possessed by detectives that induces a sense of unease among young women. Furthermore, vampires exhibit a speech pattern reminiscent of detectives, concluding their sentences with a subdued vocal tone. That is precisely why vampires possess an extraordinary power of attraction towards women.

Anklets can evoke a strong sense of sensuality and allure when worn by a woman.

It is undeniable that ankle bracelets evoke sensuality in women throughout the day. Present her with ankle bracelets as a means of eliciting her sensual inclinations towards you. Anklets will not only maintain her sensuality, but also evoke continuous thoughts of you throughout her day. Ankle bracelets serve as a highly effective means of captivating a woman's attention, devoid of physical contact.

Instruct her to don attire in a crimson hue.

The color red possesses a biological appeal that is universally attractive. A woman experiences significant revitalization upon adorning a dress of the color red, as it is symbolically associated with the powerful emotion of love.

To evoke her sexual sensations, kindly request your partner to don a crimson-colored gown. Consider presenting her with a crimson lingerie set or a scarlet swimsuit. Even the most modest woman can be readily captivated by a red garment or present, as the vibrant color red elicits sensual sentiments within a woman, thus imbuing her with a seductive allure.

Be A Handyman.

It can be more effectively engaging a woman when one assumes the role of a skilled handyman. The majority of males depend on external sources rather than proactively initiating action themselves. They are rendered incapable of performing essential tasks on their own. Therefore, women often avoid being with them.

Conversely, a handyman generates sexual energy attributable to his proactive nature. He attends to various household maintenance tasks, including repairing items, washing his vehicle, preparing elaborate meals, mowing the lawn, and brewing coffee, among other responsibilities. He has a strong inclination towards taking proactive steps, and he emanates his sense of masculinity. A woman experiences an uplifting aura of sexual energy in the company of a skilled tradesperson.

Dominate Her Mind.

A method of enticing a woman without physical contact is to exert mental dominance over her. Women have historically been drawn to men who exercise mental dominance, possess a compelling sense of humor, and engage them with fascinating narratives. If your aim is to completely captivate a woman's mindset, then it would be beneficial for you to acquire proficiency in the craft of narrative discourse.

The mingling of intrigue and enjoyment within your dialog evokes sensual sensations in a woman.

To elicit sexual desires in a woman, amusing her with engaging narratives, piquing her intellectual curiosity, and maintaining a sense of originality would be advisable. When you elicit laughter from a woman while simultaneously nurturing her intrigue with your narratives, you effortlessly stimulate her sexual desires towards you.

Please be advised that failing to ignite curiosity may result in relegating yourself to the category of her friend. Maintaining a sense of inquisitiveness is paramount in ensuring that women remain alert and engaged at all times.

Boys make women laugh. Conversely, adults elicit the sexual inclinations of women through curiosity and amusement.

Seductive Body Language.

A lady possesses the ability to promptly perceive and interpret the non-verbal cues conveyed by your physical behavior. The majority of the counsel often emphasizes fundamental nonverbal cues, whereas a woman astutely observes and takes note of your every action. It can be exceedingly challenging for an ordinary individual to conceal their true persona and project seductive nonverbal cues.

If you desire to captivate a woman through the art of seductive non-verbal communication, allow me to offer you some advice that will prove beneficial throughout your lifetime.

Do not engage in rapid head nodding. It demonstrates a sense of enthusiasm and a lack of patience. You exhibit the demeanor of an impulsive adolescent, rather than embodying the traits of a mature man.

Keep your eyebrows relaxed. When you exhibit confident nonverbal cues, you tend to neglect allowing your eyebrows to relax. When a woman observes the subtle elevation of your eyebrows, she promptly discerns your discomfort and discerns you are endeavoring to conceal your inner exhilaration.

Your countenance exudes a captivating charm that greatly appeals to the fairer sex. Have you ever contemplated the factors contributing to Johnny Depp's remarkable appeal to the female population? This is due to his aesthetically pleasing facial features and his ability to evoke strong emotional reactions from women through his facial expressions. Your eyebrows play a vital role in enhancing the appeal of your facial expressions. Therefore, adjust your eyebrows and correct your facial expressions in order to captivate a woman.

How to initiate physical contact with a woman starting from the initial introduction until the moment you both engage in a sexual encounter.

When acquiring the skill of physical contact with a woman, it is imperative to prioritize two fundamental aspects. Firstly, it is crucial for one to always maintain a state of complete ease when engaging in physical contact with women. Secondly, one must ensure that every instance of physical touch is executed in a manner that elicits a sense of absolute comfort from the woman involved.

The crucial aspect of comprehending these two essential elements is that when you make physical contact with a woman and she recognizes that your touch is completely instinctive and enjoyable to you, not only will she begin to place greater trust in you, but she will also develop a strong sense of ease in reciprocating physical contact with you. The reason why she will place greater trust in you is because it has been extensively tested and proven that when you engage in natural and enjoyable conversation with a woman, it is highly probable that she will soon begin to subconsciously perceive you as an authority or expert in the topic you are discussing with her.

Once you have successfully established a sense of comfort and trust with her, your focus should shift towards employing appropriate tactile gestures that align with the corresponding mental state across the three distinct phases of interaction: attraction, rapport, and seduction. Next, I will now proceed to divulge the three sequential measures to establish physical contact with a woman, commencing from the initial encounter and extending until the moment of intimacy is reached.

Utilize manual gestures to establish a connection that spans the divide between refraining from physical contact with her and commencing to engage in touch.

When acquiring the skill of initiating physical contact with a woman during the initial stages of an interaction, it is imperative to ensure that you adhere to the following two crucial guidelines: firstly, it is essential to master the art of using hand gestures in a manner that does not involve making physical contact with the woman, in order to establish a connection between abstaining from touch and eventually initiating touch; secondly, it is vital to learn the appropriate techniques for touching her without causing any discomfort or distress. Following this, I will proceed to provide you with a comprehensive set of sequential guidelines pertaining to the seamless transition from refraining to make physical contact with her to initiating gradual physical contact with finesse.

Prior to initiating physical contact with an unfamiliar woman, it is imperative to ascertain her complete comfort with such tactile interactions.

The most prudent approach to transitioning from refraining any physical contact with her to initiating physical contact is to employ appropriate hand gestures. Incorporating hand gestures into your interactions can effectively aid in overcoming any initial barriers women may have towards physical contact.

Your hand gestures serve the purpose of skillfully navigating into her personal space while abstaining from physical contact at present, while simultaneously subtly signaling your likelihood of touching her in the near future. Once she develops a sense of ease and trust with you encroaching upon her personal boundaries without physical contact, you may then proceed to initiating physical contact.

Allow me to provide you with instructions regarding the course of action. While engaging in conversation with the woman, attempt to subtly maneuver one of your hands in her vicinity, allowing for a seamless entrance into her personal space. You simulate the action of touching her without physically making physical contact with her. Simply position your hand in close proximity to hers, as if you were about to make physical contact. It is advisable to handle the situation with caution and take slow measures, as moving too swiftly may elicit a reaction causing her to instinctively shield or defend herself. I propose that you repetitively perform the aforementioned hand gesture until it becomes evident that she has attained a state of complete ease with it. After observing her full comfort with your hand gestures, you may proceed with physical contact.

I will now proceed to demonstrate the appropriate methodologies for initiating physical contact with a woman at each of the distinct phases of interpersonal engagement: namely, attraction, establishment of rapport, and eventual seduction.

Gently caress her playfully for a brief moment during the initial phase of attraction.

When engaging with a lady during the phase of mutual interest, it is essential to ensure that any physical contact is brief, lasting no more than 1-3 seconds. This is precisely why certain esteemed seduction practitioners prefer to refer to this type of touch as a transient touch. During the stage of attraction, it is important for your touch to evoke a sense of playfulness and lightness on her skin. This approach aims to generate a strong attraction towards you, as you touch her in a manner that conveys your potential interest without appearing overly needy or desperate. It is imperative that, at this juncture, you adopt a lighthearted mindset.

The portions of the female anatomy that are deemed suitable to make physical contact with during the phase of attraction encompass her upper extremity, specifically the outer region of her arm, as well as her shoulders and upper dorsal area. For instance, you may consider embracing a friendly gesture by casually placing your arm around her shoulder. However, please exercise caution and refrain from encircling her neck with your arm as it is important to respect that many women may find this act discomforting.

Gently and tenderly make contact with her for a duration of 3-5 seconds during the phase of establishing a close connection, assuming the role of her closest companion.

It is advisable to adopt the mentality of being a woman's closest companion when engaging with her at the stage of establishing rapport, as this aids in the cultivation of trust and a sense of ease.

In this context, it is imperative to shed the playful mindset that was previously embraced during the phase of attraction. It is also imperative to exercise caution and refrain from hastily entertaining thoughts of engaging in sexual activity with the woman while in the phase of building rapport. You aim to project an attitude of independence and self-sufficiency, displaying a complete lack of desire or neediness to obtain anything from her. At this juncture, your primary objective should be to establish acquaintance with her.

In the stage of building interpersonal connection, it is advisable to establish physical contact with the intention of conveying a sense of intimacy and trust, as if confiding something unique and exclusive to the individual. It is essential to be prepared to provide emotional support in the event that she is experiencing sadness or struggling with any difficulties. It is imperative to promote a sense of acceptance in her by demonstrating a comprehensive understanding of both her personal circumstances and her current state of affairs. Even if she expresses a preference for occasionally engaging in physical discipline with her small dogs, it would be advisable for you to demonstrate your comprehension and acceptance of her viewpoint.

The appropriate form of physical contact to employ during the phase of establishing a harmonious connection is a persistent touch. This particular form of contact has a duration of approximately 3 to 5 seconds. At this juncture, your tactile sensation should possess a notably gentle and compassionate quality.

The body areas of the woman that are deemed acceptable for contact during a state of connect are her hands, lower back, and face.

Allow me to offer you a brief indication of caution. When making contact with the woman's hands, it is appropriate to maintain gentle physical contact for a duration of 3 to 5 seconds, while refraining from clasping or gripping them.

The rationale behind limiting physical contact with the woman to a maximum of 5 seconds during the rapport-building phase is rooted in the objective of inciting her desire for further tactile interaction. This endearing approach essentially aids in creating a sense of comfort and readiness in her, preparing her for the subsequent phase of seduction, all while minimizing any potential resistance on her part.

The manner in which you would make physical contact with her during the stage of rapport is such that, for instance, you would delicately push and sweep her hair away from her face. Additionally, you have the option to gently place your hand on the nape of her neck and gradually trace your fingers upwards along the back of her head. This poignant technique has demonstrated its efficacy when transitioning from the stage of establishing rapport to the stage of seduction.

The aforementioned tactful approach can be employed by expressing something along the lines of: "May I briefly attempt this technique to ascertain its sensation?" Subsequently, place one of your hands at the base of the woman's neck and ascend along her neck, ensuring that your fingers face the crown of her head. Therefore, you would gently glide your fingertips along her neck as if you were preparing to grasp her hair. Subsequently, seizing a handful of her hair would be done at the root of her hair. Subsequently, one may proceed by gently guiding her head in a backward and downward motion in order to encourage her to elevate it.

Here's an important warning. I highly recommend that you solely engage in the act of grasping and pulling the hair during the final stage of establishing a strong bond.

Caress her with strength and tenderness to your heart's content during the phase of seduction.

In the phase of attracting her, it is advisable to engage in physical contact that conveys strength and dominance. Your physical contact should exude strength and masculinity while also exhibiting tenderness, as it is imperative to ensure that she is not subjected to any form of harm. To ensure that you do not cause her any harm, it is advisable to combine a touch of lightheartedness with your masculine strength. However, it is crucial to maintain a sustained level of sexual arousal during this phase, as any abrupt decrease in your own state of arousal can swiftly dissipate the woman's sexual state as well, ultimately terminating the engagement.

In the context of romantic pursuit, it is advisable to ensure that physical contact is initiated in a manner that conveys a strong sense of intimacy and sensuality. Your touch ought to evoke an intense sense of desire within the woman, as your intention is to engender a profound feeling of desirability within her.

Throughout the phase of seduction, it is advisable to maintain a consistent level of tactility. The consistent physical contact indicates your ability to sustain touch on a specific area of her body for an extended duration.

Your tactile experience should encompass not just a substantial and masculine strength, but also a conspicuous weightiness in the palm. The phrase 'palm heavy' denotes the action of smoothly transitioning from touching her lower back to touching her legs by consistently gliding the palm of your hand from the lower back area, along the entirety of her buttocks, all the way down to her legs. Put simply, there is no necessity to disengage your hand from her lower back to proceed with relocating it onto her legs or any other desired area of her body that you wish to contact subsequently.

It is highly advisable to refrain from raising one's hand while transitioning from one area of physical contact with a person to another, as doing so poses the potential risk of abruptly causing the person to lose their state of sexual arousal. If she abruptly ceases her state of sexual arousal, the game will reach its conclusion. It is of utmost importance to apply a delicate and gentle touch with the palm while engaging in the process of seduction.

Here's an important note. Ensure that you refrain from issuing an apology to the woman for any physical contact made in a specific manner, provided that such contact was executed appropriately and within the appropriate context of the interaction. I highly recommend against apologizing to her for it due to the potential implications it may have. Not only could she subconsciously perceive you as an individual with significant insecurities and questionable intentions, but she may also vehemently reject your advances.

Here is why she perceives your apologies as unattractive: whenever you apologize to the woman for something that does not necessitate an apology, she will immediately view you as a highly vulnerable individual who lacks confidence in himself and his emotions.

Regarding the female body regions that are deemed suitable for contact during the phase of seduction, it goes without saying that you may initiate physical contact with any part of her body, as long as you ensure that your actions do not cause her any harm.

What To Avoid: The Off-Putting Factors

There are no strict guidelines when it comes to engaging in explicit language. Nevertheless, I have compiled a comprehensive list for your perusal, pertaining to the generally disadvised elements when engaging in risqué discourse.

Don't:

Do not exert yourself to engage in explicit conversation. Individuals, particularly those with whom we have established partnerships, possess an inherent ability to accurately discern the genuineness of our behavior. The primary source of arousal stems from your partner perceiving your genuine enthusiasm and engagement in the situation.

Please refrain from using vulgar or inappropriate language if it causes discomfort. Certain women find the term "C*nt" to be highly off-putting. Please focus on using words that are either neutral to you or ones that you find stimulating.

Exercise restraint in engaging in excessive explicit conversation, particularly if you detect that your partner exhibits signs of unease or discomfort. Engage in a subtle exchange with them and affirm their words by expressing how greatly their provocative conversation is arousing you.

Avoid introducing explicit sexual conversation prematurely, especially if you have only been on a few dates and are uncertain about your partner's level of sexual conservatism.

Avoid mentioning the size of someone's unit, particularly if it is smaller, unless they believe you lack experience with larger units and you can successfully deceive them. There exist alternative methods by which one may employ verbal expression to instill a sense of positivity within him.

It is advised to refrain from discussing your unconventional preferences or fetishes, such as desires involving urination, during the initial stages of a conversation.

It is advisable not to engage in explicit discussions regarding violence, such as discussing desires to choke, in the context of intimate conversations, unless the exploration of violence-related fantasies has been previously addressed and mutually agreed upon through a prior dialogue with one's partner.

It is advisable not to indicate to a person that you are about to experience orgasm, if you do not wish for them to reach climax immediately. It is widely understood that men may reach orgasm more quickly when informed of imminent climax, such as by saying phrases like "I'm going to ejaculate" or "Please continue, I'm reaching orgasm." To prolong the experience, it is advisable not to indicate that climax is imminent unless the intention is to bring about immediate ejaculation and cessation of activity.

Do not make the assumption that his gender automatically correlates with unpleasant behavior. It can occasionally be necessary to gradually introduce men and women to the concept of engaging in provocative or explicit conversation. An individual might initially be unaccustomed to their partner engaging in explicit conversations, but as they actively participate, they gradually discover that it enhances their sexual arousal. Commence the process by gradually transitioning through the sequential procedures elucidated in the subsequent chapter.

Chapter Four

Strategies for Gradually Introducing Erotic Conversation

Females are frequently brought up with the expectation of displaying reserved and courteous behavior. Employing vocal expression provides liberation and can be highly gratifying for women. Expressing oneself verbally during intimate moments can enhance and enrich one's sexual experiences. It entails utilizing one's vocal expressions to foster a heightened and mutually enriching experience between oneself and their partner. Explicit conversations extend beyond mere imitation of adult film dialogues and suggestive vocal tones. It entails articulating your own experiences, as well as the envisioned shared experiences, with your partner.

To gradually incorporate explicit language into a conversation, you can effortlessly utilize verbal expression to articulate or signify pleasure. Employ terms such as "increased intensity," "enhanced force," or "accelerated pace" to convey your desires. If you wish to gradually acclimate yourself, you may initiate with fundamental gratification. Initially, through vocal expressions of discomfort or distress, followed by verbal requests for increased intensity, heightened exertion, or accelerated pace.

An additional suggestion for developing proficiency in engaging in explicit language is to peruse written works of erotica. You have the opportunity to peruse the initial pages of any book without charge, enabling you to ascertain if it aligns with your personal preferences.

In addition, it is also possible to recount a recollection or experience from your past. Communicate with them the intense heat that was prevailing and convey your sensations during that scorching encounter. Discuss your imaginative desires.

Regarding the topic of engaging in explicit conversation, for those who lack experience, it is not uncommon to feel uneasy. Articulating one's thoughts with precision can prove to be a challenging endeavor.

Initiate the conversation by expressing my anticipation for engaging in a passionate and intimate connection with you.

What thoughts occupy your mind during a sexual encounter? You bring me immense pleasure in our intimate connection. I appreciate the sensation of your presence within me." "I perceive the pulsating sensation from within me." "I sense the gripping sensation of your intimacy.

Women want to be craved after. Women desire to be desired. They desire to experience sensuality. Communicate to them the impact they are having on your state of rigidity. Express to them the impact that their legs have on your emotions. Every woman possesses inherent beauty and deserves sincere appreciation for the allure and impact they exude upon others. One can exhibit significant creativity and gradually develop a more intense approach.

Once you gradually introduce intimate language into your conversation, you will observe that thoughts and expressions will effortlessly come forth.

Chapter 3

Guidelines for Appropriate and Inappropriate Conversation

Mastering the art of sensual language is a skill that should be cultivated by all individuals. It presents a valuable opportunity to arouse one's partner and enhance intimacy within the confines of the bedroom. In any event, the task at hand is challenging, and there is no definitive method to accomplish it as each relationship is unique and each woman has varying preferences. There exists a minimal distinction between explicit language and repugnant discourse, and achieving equality in this matter is difficult to ascertain. In order to facilitate the articulation of appropriate dialogue, we engaged in conversation with a select group of women proficient in the art of candid communication on matters of a sensual nature. Through this interaction, we ascertained the existence of a set of universally accepted guidelines and principles.

Make an effort to abstain from employing derogatory language. I don't care for being known as a prostitute. Please refrain from making any indirect references to my female anatomy.

Phrases such as "cunt" can be deemed inappropriate and offensive. Such words are disruptive and can be seen as disrespectful. Irrespective of the absence of malicious intentions on your part, we perceive the utterances.

Similar sentiments are commonly evoked by such expressions, leading to an inherent inclination towards unfavorability.

contrarily. It completely removes us from our existing state, separate from everything else. An overall dampener of enthusiasm, occasionally

hostile.

Please inform me if you find me physically appealing. I greatly appreciate it when, during an intimate encounter, a man gently lifts my body upwards and

Brings me down and indicates that I am enticing. It enhances my aura, eliciting a delightful sensation and immediately...

Compels me to take action in order to elicit a similar reaction from him.

Please refrain from directing me towards tranquility. When I was having intercourse with an ex and he was experiencing difficulty

While climbing to the summit, I inquired, "Are you in a satisfactory state?" to which he responded with a hushed "Shhh" in order to concentrate. It was so

Rudely, he gave the impression of potentially participating in intimate activities with an inflatable figurine and overall conducting himself inappropriately.

fulfilled. Undoubtedly, he failed to conclude.

Please inform me if you require assistance throughout the night. Regardless of our endeavors, nothing seems to render a youthful lady

I experience a sense of superiority when considering the notion that the gentleman in question ought to persist in such endeavors. This signifies that he has achieved satisfaction, and

As long as my preference aligns with it, it will necessitate my persistence.

Please consider using a condom as a precautionary measure. No matter how fervently you endeavor to depict its allure, should we not...

Given our limited familiarity, I do not possess any inclination to engage in an intimate act with you without any protection. Firstly, considering the fact that I do not...

I am aware of everyone's well-being, and secondly, considering the unappealing nature of that statement.

Do command. The substantial impact on our lives as women pertains to the management of situations and the provision of care.

Amongst our fellow persons, it is comforting to have someone assume authority and manage our affairs, thus providing a sense of relief. So feel

Kindly inform me of your requirements or preferences. A person who is assertive and expressive is attractive.

It substantially diminishes the workload required to attend to other tasks.

Please refrain from being condescending. With that being stated, I was informed by an individual in the past that I was committing an error

Moreover, I met instantaneous death. I experienced a profound sense of inadequacy, and I have no desire to

Continue participating in intimate encounters with the person who evoked such emotions within me. Should you desire my assistance

Present an alternative suggestion in a forthright manner, without implying any disregard or severity towards my current approach.

Kindly address me by my name. It substantiates his presence and engagement in the particular gathering, evoking a profound sense of assurance within me.

I represent a distinct persona, characterized by my youth. It is quite warm, especially when he softly utters my name into my ear while he-

Kindly inform me about the immense satisfaction it provides. Sex serves as a potent medium for elucidating the underlying dynamics of human relationships, encapsulating the truth residing at the core of each connection

The exchange of names strongly reinforces the notion that we are currently united in this moment.

Endeavor to avoid becoming too specialized. The terms penis and vagina were used in reference to the specialist's clinic, rather than

the room. That is a guaranteed success in the realm of sexual activity. In the event that I required to create a comfortable environment

I would consult my gynecologist in collaboration with my specialist.

Please inform me of the extent to which I feel or experience a sensation of greatness. "Basic expressions of admiration greatly resonate with young women, although a more nuanced approach is preferred, such as uttering, '

If we consistently iterate phrases such as 'You possess an immense level of physical allure/charm/grace,' the essence behind the words could gradually diminish, ultimately resulting in a mere platitudinous exchange.

Presume that you have exhausted all your points of discussion. Should you

happen to find my taste or sensation
pleasing, kindly express it. It may sound

Although it may appear unconventional
in your thoughts, we derive pleasure
from its expression.

Enhancing Intimate Connection: Tantra Practices And Therapeutic Massages To Cultivate Sexual Satisfaction In Relationships

Having its roots in what is currently known as modern India, Tantra is estimated to be at least 5000-7000 years old, predating and exerting influence on both Hinduism and Buddhism.

Numerous religious doctrines maintain that one can only attain either physical gratification or spiritual enlightenment, but not both simultaneously.

According to Tantra, there is a fundamental contradiction as they perceive that the culmination of our spiritual development relies on the attainment of physical and sensual gratification. The absence of either one would consequently render the other unattainable.

Tantrics hold the belief that by engaging in bodily practices, one can effectively eliminate accumulated impurities, thus facilitating healing and fostering a reintroduction to the encompassing spiritual energy. A fundamental tenet of Tantra lies in its conviction regarding the existence of a spirit or energetic potency, asserting that both the cosmos as a whole and each individual within it are imbued with this same vitality. Significantly, adherents of Tantra hold the belief that any suppression of this vital energy results in an imbalance and detriment to our well-being.

Tantra opposes the restrictive, moralistic, self-renouncing ethical principles advocated by various religions, wherein our physical and sensory desires are met with feelings of guilt, further guilt, suppression, refusal, and penalization. In instances where consideration is directed towards physiological requirements, it is commonly oriented towards prevention, such as the avoidance of ailments or unintended conception. Insufficient emphasis is placed on the cultivation and enrichment of our physical sensuality, with no guidance provided on how to fully embrace and appreciate it.

According to tantrics, in order to develop as fully-realized individuals, it is necessary to address and remove obstructions that exist within our physical and psychic systems. The majority of individuals embrace the concept of physical systems. We are all aware of the existence of physiological organs such as the Liver, Heart, and Stomach. However, have we considered the presence of psychic systems? Controversial though it may be, it is nonetheless widely acknowledged among most prominent religious doctrines that the essence of our existence transcends the mere confines of our physical form.

Tantric practitioners hold the belief that a potent spiritual force, known as the base chakra, is located in the area between our lower extremities. Upon being released, it ascends through our system. Our knowledge remains restricted when it is in a dormant state, but when activated, it enables the organic progression of spiritual growth that we ought to be undergoing.

This essential life force, known as Kundalini, is nourished through conduits referred to as Meridians. Any form of obstruction hampers the smooth flow of energy, similar to how a kinked hose-pipe restricts the supply of water.

Numerous individuals uphold the notion that one tangible expression of the "Life Energy" is the Aura. The topic of whether it is an aura, characterized by its quasi-religious connotations, or simply electricity, remains a subject of intense discussion. Recent scientific studies have provided evidence supporting the existence of a widely distributed electromagnetic field surrounding the human body. Additionally, these studies indicate that all bodily tissues and organs, including the Heart and the Brain, generate their own distinct electrical impulses. Is there a connection between this relatively recent research and the Tantric belief in the Chakra system, which depicts whirling wheels of energy that spiral throughout our body, merging the various aspects and levels of our existence? According to Tantrics, when these energy centers are in proper functioning order, so too are we. In a similar vein to the Meridians, external factors such as lifestyle, conditioning, guilt, and diet serve as impediments that hinder their optimal functionality. When they become obstructed, we experience a decline in our performance and lack energy.

Tantrics and some contemporary therapies posit that we possess numerous obstructions of this nature and argue that traumatic experiences, such as recollected sorrow, distress, humiliation, physical or emotional mistreatment, persist ensconced within our corporeal form. The repercussions of this initial obstruction persist throughout our lifespan, adversely affecting our overall welfare and vitality. It is conceivable that we may even experience physical constriction in our throats due to childhood indoctrination against expressing emotions through crying or raising our voices. Our pelvis can become inflexible as a result of our efforts to suppress our sexual urges. It is possible that our anal sphincter has become constricted and remains constricted as a consequence of our previous, and often overlooked, efforts to suppress feelings of anger.

The Massage

Tantrics employ various techniques to "restore" our body, firmly believing in its profound significance to our overall wellness. One example of this is massage, as it is believed that massage and Tantric techniques can effectively dismantle obstructions and eliminate them, resulting in healing and restoration of the body.

What sets Tantric massage apart from other forms of massage are the distinct techniques it employs, which may be familiar in other massage practices.

I would like to propose five suggestions;

Therapeutic masseurs prioritize the direct physical benefits, whereas sensualists view pleasure as a distinct objective. Tantrics hold the belief that pleasure serves as the conduit to spirituality—a means to an ultimate goal.

In the practice of Tantra, we express generosity without expecting any form of compensation, and we accept without feeling obliged to provide something in return.

It can be regarded as a means of receiving and bestowing sensual gratification, devoid of any requirement for engaging in explicit sexual acts.

There are no externally imposed barriers in terms of location, subject, and methodology of touching. The only obstacles present are the ones that we, as conscientious adults, have consciously chosen to have in place. If the agreement permits comprehensive exploration of your partner's entire physique, both you and they may discover novel, entirely unforeseen sources of pleasure. A considerable number of individuals from Western cultures often exhibit a strong focus on matters pertaining to the genitals. We often neglect the remaining 95% of our physique, a substantial portion of which possesses the potential to elicit diverse yet similarly exquisite reactions. Through this approach, Tantra perpetuates the sense of freedom that individuals experience when they come to the realization that touch is an inherent and reciprocally fulfilling interaction.

There exist specific methods for both respiration and manipulation of specific regions of the physique, such as the Chakras or reproductive organs, which are characteristic of the Tantra tradition, as well as the Chinese Tao.

Tantra embodies a release, an indulgent passage that has the potential to yield remarkable elation. Pursuing transparency and integrity, this approach to the body is both uplifting and characterized by discipline. It facilitates - promotes - an unrestricted opportunity to engage, explore, appreciate, and openly revel in our physical being in a manner that individuals in Western societies might alternatively find disconcerting, invigorating, embarrassing, and, potentially, ultimately emancipating. The outcomes of adopting such openness, coupled with its emphasis on the significance of the process rather than the outcome, can be remarkable for individuals who are accustomed to focusing solely on the conclusion (for example, ejaculation in men, which it discourages, and if she is fortunate, orgasm for women). It provides ample opportunity for us to direct our attention towards our partner and the diverse range of sensations their body experiences. Tantra does not have many taboos, if any, as long as whatever is done is carried out with mutual respect and voluntary consent, although this condition is of utmost importance. In the practice of Tantra, the utilization of power dynamics, coercion, emotional manipulation, or exploitation is deemed unacceptable...

Deu to all the previously mentioned factors, Tantra is exceptionally apt for a massage.

Technique for Sensual Massage for Men

For centuries, the practice of Tantric sexuality and massage has not only served as a means of cultivating closer bonds between partners, but has also proven instrumental in fostering profound connections with one's significant other, oneself, and the broader universe. By partaking in the practice of Tantric massage or male erotic massage, individuals can explore the advantages of engaging in intimate sessions with a cherished partner who possesses a deep understanding of the principles underlying male genital massage. There is a commonly held belief that Tantric massage is primarily focused on sexual stimulation, but it should be noted that it encompasses a broader aspect. While it does incorporate sexual elements, the underlying goal is centered around self-healing, personal exploration, and the utilization of sexual energy in the context of self-discovery and intimacy with one's partner.

Tantric massage is a sacred encounter that pertains to the spiritual aspects of Tantra. Indeed, the term Tantra signifies the pursuit of individual advancement within a realm of enjoyable existence. By means of this massage, you can initiate an unprecedented sense of enjoyment, embracing the transformative essence of Tantra. Its deeply spiritual nature will provide profound enlightenment to the universe, oneself, and the encompassing surroundings. There exist various methodologies for undertaking Tantric male massage, often incorporating gentle hand movements along the head and shaft of the penis with the intent of prolonging pleasure for both the masseuse and the recipient of the sensual male massage. Throughout the duration of the massage, maintaining a consistent focus on gentle, delicate fingertip manipulation is essential to ensure the desired experience is achieved during the Tantric massage.

It is crucial to bear in mind that the objective is not mere sexual gratification through Tantric massage, but rather to cultivate a profoundly heightened connection between oneself and their significant other. During our previous discussion, we deliberated on the advantages of engaging in sexual activities. Although Tantric massage does not involve sexual intercourse, it is rooted in harnessing sexual energy. Utilizing sexual energy in the context of Tantric massage can yield significant benefits for the physical well-being of individuals.

Whether it is accomplished through the modality of sexual energy healing or by means of the tranquility and stress reduction that accompanies Tantric massage. The remarkable aspect of Tantric male massage lies not only in its pleasurable sensation, but also in its extensive array of health and stress-reducing advantages, which extend to both the recipient and the provider of the massage.

Both individuals will be prepared to engage in an extraordinary intimate encounter that will foster a sense of closeness through the process of exploring their partner and self-discovery.

By applying therapeutic manipulation to the genital region of the individual and facilitating their exploration of heightened states of sensual gratification, the masseuse assists in elevating the individual's cognitive state to an enhanced level, enabling them to attain tranquility, rejuvenation, and enhanced resilience for navigating their surroundings. It is imperative to grasp the advantages associated with Tantric male massage, while also avoiding any misconceptions or conflation with sexual activities. Sexual energy does play a role, but it is important to clarify that Tantric massage, in essence, is not synonymous with sexual activity; rather, it represents an exploration of oneself, in the presence of a beloved partner. If you contemplate engaging in the practice of Tantric massage on an individual, you are in essence introducing them to an entirely unexplored realm of experience, facilitating their personal discovery and mutual exploration with the utilization of the Tantric approach to male massage.

Essential Suggestions for Heat Therapy - Tantric Bodywork

Guidelines for Therapeutic Techniques: Tantric Massage

Prior to delving further into the intricacies of this massage technique, it is imperative for us to apprehend that Tantric massage possesses exceptional characteristics which render it distinct and highly exclusive. Similar to other types of massage, Tantra massage offers its own distinct advantages. What particularly captivates me is the emphasis placed on our emotional and spiritual well-being rather than solely on our physical health.

Unfortunately, it's not that common and, therefore, not readily available just everywhere due to the specialist skills and training involved. The individual responsible for offering such massage services must possess expert proficiency in both fundamental and advanced tenets of Tantra and meditation.

The Tantric massage session commences with traditional Tantric rituals and a period of meditation, designed to cultivate awareness of the Chakras and establish a profound spiritual connection with the entirety of the universe.

It is important to always bear in mind that this type of massage is not intended to alleviate the stresses and strains that our bodies have endured, to facilitate muscle relaxation, or to prioritize our physical well-being. The practice of Tantric massage induces a profound awakening of latent mystical energy, fostering a state of complete alignment between the physical body and the spiritual essence, synchronized harmoniously with the cosmic realm.

The practice of Tantric massage incorporates gentle, sensual, and deliberate movements designed to facilitate the flow of energy and enhance the body's receptiveness to an alternative state of being. It is recommended to apply moderate pressure along the sides of the spine to ensure the effectiveness of the massage. However, for the most part, it is advised to limit the pressure to a lighter touch and to focus on movements inspired by the natural flow of energy through the body, particularly the traditional upward movement starting from the base of the spine.

I advise against underestimating the significance of this type of massage. Don't play at it. A substantial amount of expertise is necessary, accompanied by a comprehensive understanding of your internal energy, before even considering the undertaking of a Tantric massage.

I am confident that the significance and advantages of a Tantric massage have been devalued due to individuals who may have experienced it without comprehending its authentic essence and the extremely refined expertise necessary to administer an authentic Tantric massage.

Meditation and the harmonious strains of music are the sole requisites for this particular form of massage. However, the music employed should possess a notable association with meditation and the cultivation of spiritual enlightenment. Music specifically intended for Tantric massage exists but is not widely available and may be challenging to locate.

While not essential, one could also opt to utilize oils and lotions, as I suppose there exists a belief that a massage would not be considered complete without their inclusion. To preserve the overall impact of this massage technique, it is advisable to refrain from utilizing fragrant oils, as they have the potential to be diverting in and of themselves.

Engage in the practice of Tantric massage with your significant other. When executed proficiently, it unquestionably enhances the levels of intimacy and fosters a more robust emotional and spiritual connection between the individuals involved.

This objective is accomplished by cultivating and nurturing the existing bond of love and trust, rather than directing attention towards sexual aspects.

Therapeutic Techniques for Manipulating Soft Tissues

The concept of Tantra encompasses a deeper significance beyond our current understanding. The genesis of this practice can be traced back to ancient India, spanning more than five millennia. Tantra revolves around the channeling of vitality and the dissemination of sensual vitality throughout the body, with less emphasis on cognitive aspects. It serves as an instigator for unveiling and embracing our emotional and sexual aspects. In the tantric tradition, sexual experiences can be likened to a strategic game of football, wherein team managers, along with the technical staff, observe and provide guidance to the players throughout the course of the game. Tantra possesses an abundance of competent instructors, advisors, and trainers to cater to its needs.

When initiating a massage, the individual who will be receiving the massage assumes a horizontal position, with the aid of pillows or any suitable material for support, while the individual who will be administering the massage assumes responsibility for carrying out the task. The unclothed individual reclining on a bed, with their genitals fully exposed, is intended to commence the activity by engaging in deep, relaxed respiration. This particular breathing technique serves as a means of achieving complete relaxation and should be implemented intermittently throughout the massage session. Massage oil is utilized, and in order to ensure the recipient breathes deeply, continuous prompting is necessary as it traverses the body.

In the context of men, the comprehensive areas to focus on would encompass the male reproductive organ, scrotum, pubic bone, g-spot, testicles, perineum, among others. Administer a complete body massage to induce an overall state of complete relaxation, followed by proceeding to apply firm pressure to the penis. Raise the object with enough care to provide a soothing sensation to the testicles; proceed to maneuver the main part horizontally, to the left, and forwards, similar to adjusting the gear lever in a motor vehicle. The aspect of speed is not a relevant component of this particular activity; the focus lies on the emotions experienced and the emanation of energy, which are currently highly valued. Gently stimulate the cranial region to promote relaxation of the nervous system and facilitate therapeutic benefits. If a person feels inclined towards ejaculation during this process, it is advisable to redirect the focus to other areas of the body. Attain the location of the g-spot if possible in order to enhance his orgasm and address his inability to regulate ejaculation. In this region, exercise caution and further alleviate any discomfort, as it is frequently uncomfortable initially.

If a woman is the recipient, commence with the exposed chest and proceed with care as she inhales deeply. Breasts are esteemed attributes, experience the warmth of affection emanating from them, handle them with care; subsequently, proceed to the abdominal region. Please proceed to the public area and refrain from approaching the vulva region in the event that it may elicit arousal. Administer a comprehensive massage to her entire body, paying close attention to her lower extremities, and carefully observe her demeanor. Determine her readiness; the allocation of sexual energy holds great significance as it is the essence of existence. The heightened morale contributes to the intricate and pleasurable nature of tantric practice.

Tantric lovemaking is a highly intricate and pleasurable practice that promotes prolonged endurance for men, enabling them to sustain the act for extended periods, possibly even throughout an entire night. Simultaneously, women experience a reinvigoration of complete orgasmic release and fulfillment. Engaging in intimate physical activity is not a mere fleeting experience, characterized by brief moments of excitement followed by slumber. Rather, it is a complex and intricate process that unfolds in its own unique way, offering complete solace and contentment to both partners involved. Establish a profound connection between affectionate emotional bond and the gratification derived from intimate experiences, as it emanates from one's deepest emotions. Intently focus your attention and experience the heightened sensory pleasure while engaging in prolonged mutual eye contact. Once prepared, let the organs come together and establish a firm connection, allowing them to experience the profound energy flowing throughout the body, reaching up to the head. Maintain your focus and experience the pleasure of the meeting of the genitalia, refraining from hastening into any actions. Engaging in sexual activity entails being fully charged and maintaining a state of stillness.

How to Indulge in an Exceptional Tantra Massage Experience

There are multiple approaches to acquiring knowledge and engaging in the practice of Tantra. Of all the methods available, tantric massage emerges as the most effective one. A comprehensive tantric massage encompasses various elements beyond the physical manipulation of tissues. Additionally, this form of massage incorporates appropriate meditation practices, tantric yoga exercises, mindful breathing techniques, deep relaxation methods, and highly efficient sexual techniques.

In contrast to other massage techniques, the practice of tantra massage necessitates the establishment of an emotional connection between the provider and the recipient. It is quite customary that an unfamiliar individual cannot fulfill someone's needs or desires in the same manner that a familiar person is capable of doing. Hence, it would be advisable to steer clear of any advertisements purporting to offer efficacious tantric massages. Proper trust and proper intimacy are the two basic things of various tantra rituals, exercises, and tantra techniques.

An individual should engage in specific actions in order to experience a beneficial tantric massage. To begin with, it is imperative that the massage is conducted within an environment that facilitates holistic relaxation for the body and mind. The location should additionally remain devoid of any disturbances. The location must be completely isolated from any form of external contact.

The surface upon which the massage would be conducted holds equal significance as the surrounding ambiance. Given that comfort and relaxation are commonly desired, a plush mattress, cushion, or even a pristine sheet can effectively serve this purpose. Towels that provide adequate support to the knees and neck are necessary. Discover the opportunity to procure premium massage oil infused with herbal extracts, known to amplify the therapeutic benefits of the massage experience. There are several additional factors that can enhance the level of relaxation achieved through tantric massage. The combination of delicately scented incense, melodic religious music, and the gentle illumination of candlelight has the undeniable ability to create a sense of enchantment.

The recipient ought to assume a prone position as the massage commences. A gentle foot massage serves as an optimal choice to initiate the commencement of the massage. Over time, the focus of the treatment should transition to the neck and shoulder region. The critical pressure points located in the neck and shoulder region have the potential to induce optimal relaxation across the entire body when subjected to appropriate massage techniques. The posterior region is the subsequent area that the masseur should direct their attention towards. Proper attention should be given to the joints and muscular regions in order to assist the recipient in alleviating all forms of stress. Once the posterior region has been fully attended to, it is expected that the recipient shall gradually rotate in the opposite direction. This will aid the masseur in attending to the anterior region.

Toddlers And Babies

It is imperative that you begin using appropriate medical terminology to refer to their respective anatomical structures, such as the penis and vulva.
It is perfectly acceptable to touch all regions of their physique, granting them the autonomy to handle their genitals amidst bathing or diaper changes.

Initiate the process of delineating the differences between males and females, such as the anatomical attribute of males possessing penises in contrast to females having vulvas.

Commence by addressing the biological functions of the different anatomical components: the male genitalia/female genitalia expels urine, while the posterior/rectum facilitates the elimination of waste (and it is acceptable to employ suitable colloquialisms, though not excessively).

There exist appropriate occasions and locations for nudity, which do not include public parks. If children assert a desire for consistent nudity, it may be necessary to establish boundaries in this regard.

In a strictly technical sense, given one's current age, this falls outside the scope of sex education. Encouraging your child to thoroughly explore their entire body will facilitate their ability to discern fundamental differences between males and females. When enumerating the various components of their anatomy, individuals can acknowledge the presence of their genitals, such as the penis or vulva, while describing their bodily functions, for instance, by stating, "Indeed, there is your penis, from which urine is expelled!" The overarching goal is for your child to develop a comfortable relationship with their entire body and to appreciate each aspect equally, devoid of any sense of shame.

The enigma surrounding the optimal approach for initiating a conversation with an unfamiliar individual remains undisclosed.

Initiating a substantial dialogue with an individual who is not part of one's usual circle of acquaintances can initially evoke feelings of unease and apprehension. Regardless of whether you possess expertise in initiating discussions or struggle with engaging in casual conversation, possessing the skill to know how and where to commence holds great importance. Kindly review these methods for initiating a conversation with an unfamiliar individual:

Adopt an optimistic approach: Approach the discussion with a positive outlook. Maintain appropriate non-verbal communication to convey your enthusiasm, such as smiling and keeping your arms uncrossed.

Inhale deeply: Inhale a series of deep breaths before commencing the conversation. This will help to reduce your heart rate and alleviate any feelings of anxiety.

Exercise caution during less conventional moments: If the individual appears preoccupied or engrossed, it is advisable to keep your conversation brief.

Accumulate information

One effective approach to initiate a discourse with an individual who is not part of a particular group is to present them with a query or a sequence of inquiries. Depending on the situation at hand, you may inquire about the weather, their lunch choices, or engage in conversation regarding shared professional responsibilities. Consider this scenario: Do you have any insight into the possibility of the organization's president delivering a speech during the opening session? Attend to their response and determine the appropriate course of action for further conversation.

Commend the unfamiliar individual.

An additional approach to initiate a conversation with someone is to offer them praise or commendation. This process predominantly fosters a delightful discourse concerning the item or feature you have commended. Consider this example: I admire your haircut. In order to facilitate further conversation, please consider posing additional inquiries, such as the place where you obtained your haircut. To stimulate the discussion, you may also inquire about where I can get a similar hairstyle.

Introduce a widely-discussed topic.

Make use of your surroundings to help you initiate a conversation with someone unfamiliar. For example, in the event that you are attending an industry gathering, kindly inquire of the person in proximity to you at the studio for their perspective on the event. If you intend to grab a meal, kindly draw the attention of the person standing nearby in the queue to your preferred selection. Here is an alternative illustration: Illustration: "Are you employed within the framework?" Yesterday, I observed that your automobile was parked in close proximity to mine."

Present yourself

A presentation serves as a direct means of initiating a conversation with an individual from outside the group or organization. It is particularly feasible if there are no other evident conversation starters to rely upon. Please find enclosed a demonstration model: Greetings, I am Andrew. "I have recently undergone a relocation and it is now essential for me to familiarize myself with all the individuals within the department." It is highly probable that the person you encounter will introduce themselves and provide additional information about their background, leading to an informal conversation.

Pose open-finished inquiries

Another effective approach to initiate a conversation with an unfamiliar individual is by inquiring open-ended questions. This system is most effective when attending a commonly shared event, where one can acquire insights about the perspectives of others. As an illustration, I have not had the opportunity to visit a notably exhilarating studio. "What observations or remarks could be made regarding your character or experiences?" Typically, the other party should respond by expressing their feelings or anecdotes about various gatherings they have participated in, thus introducing additional topics for discussion.

Ensure that you remain informed about the latest advancements

Recent advancements are extraordinary conversation starters. It is advisable to avoid discussing political matters in case you and the unfamiliar individual hold contrasting viewpoints. Examine topics such as a local community event, or inquire about a recently published literary work or a recently released motion picture. Allow me to present you with an example: Have you observed that the annual Occasion Celebration is scheduled to commence in one week's time? I typically derive pleasure from leisurely walking and observing the decorations."

Extend an offer of assistance

Should you happen to observe an individual who is struggling with a particular task, offering your assistance serves as a commendable approach to initiate a conversation. Depending on the location and context of the interaction, you may employ a phrase similar to this: May I offer assistance in transporting that container for you? By any chance, are you unfamiliar with the structure?"

Present an intriguing fact

This method is most effective in situations where your intriguing fact directly correlates. When employed appropriately, this method can prove to be highly effective in engaging an individual in conversation. I would like to propose a model for your consideration: Were you already aware, to some extent, that elevators are the most secure means of transportation?"

Request their viewpoint

Consider seeking the perspective of an impartial individual in order to initiate a dialogue. This is an exceptional approach if you are situated elsewhere or aiming to locate pens within the inventory storage of your organization. This example demonstrates the proper way to utilize this.

approach: Which one of these highlighters is your preferred choice? Normally, I tend to employ these yellow ones, although the wax ones appear to be quite intriguing!"

Request lunch counsel

A feasible approach to initiate a conversation with an unfamiliar individual is to inquire about their preferred dining establishment. This is particularly beneficial in the event that you find yourself in an elevator or waiting for a taxi or public transportation, given that it offers an opportunity for expedient conversations. For instance, you may inquire about preferred dining options in the vicinity. I frequently conduct my work activities at the office located on Fifth Road, thereby piquing my interest in this particular area. The individuals possessing unique knowledge are likely to share their top-rated dining establishments, and they may even extend an invitation for you to join them for lunch.

Provide feedback on a widely-shared online video

Viral recordings hold considerable efficacy as a communicative tool. Numerous individuals engage in viewing recordings during their leisure hours or become aware of them through acquaintances or colleagues. If you decide to utilize this system, ensure that the video you observe is suitable for the professional setting. Presented below is an exemplar: Have you had the opportunity to glimpse the visual recording of the juvenile dozing off within the receptacle of frozen yogurt? Ideally, this will engender a discourse regarding other captivating recordings or topics of mainstream culture.

Be direct

In numerous instances, initiating a conversation by explicitly stating your intentions or desires is often the most effective approach. For example, in the event that you find yourself disoriented, kindly inquire about directions. To partake in a midday meal with another individual, clearly convey your intention. Allow me to present an alternative proposition: On this momentous occasion, being my initial day, I am bereft of any knowledge pertaining to the ideal location to partake in a midday repast. Could you potentially envisage any difficulties if I were to accompany you?

Request help

Seeking assistance is an effective approach to initiating a conversation. Depending on the situation, it may be necessary for you to seek assistance from a specific individual rather than anyone nearby. Consider this scenario: As I have not operated from this office before, I am unfamiliar with the functioning mechanisms involved. Do you anticipate any difficulties in assisting me?

Analyze typical hobbies or pastimes.

In specific instances, it is indeed apparent that there exists a common interest between yourself and an individual external to your circle. Employ the indicator that you perceive as an initial point for the conversation. For instance, I have observed that you also support our local basketball team. I had the opportunity to attend a sporting event last week. How about yourself? Acquiring knowledge about your new acquaintance and exchanging information about oneself typically leads to the discovery of shared interests. Focus on these specific topics and discuss them in detail; one cannot predict when new information will be unearthed. Furthermore, you may find another companion with whom to indulge in this particular hobby. If you happen to lack common interests, there is no need to worry or become anxious. It is important to remember that not everyone you encounter in life will ultimately become your closest companion. Congratulations for making it this far in the discussion!

Provide an insightful observation

Another method of initiating a conversation with a person who is not familiar to you is to make a comment concerning the surrounding environment or a shared topic of interest."

The situation in which you find yourself. This technique is most effective when there is a specific aspect to comment on, such as: I notice that you also have a preference for employing the handset instead of a headset. This type of comment allows individuals from outside the immediate situation to express their own perspectives on the matter.

Observe a prevalent characteristic

Employ this protocol when you are confident that both parties involved possess a mutually satisfactory level of excellence. Engaging in a discourse centered around a shared attribute is often a remarkable approach to cultivating an immediate rapport. Consider

Regarding this particular model, I noticed your endorsement with your left hand - coincidentally, I happen to be left-handed as well! When intriguing qualities are present, a significant number of individuals value engaging in discussions regarding the affiliation.

Inquire about their previous encounter

Gaining insights into their expertise through engaging inquiring is a professional and hospitable approach to initiating a conversation. Consider this illustration: Welcome to the cohort! From whence did you originate prior to accompanying us to this place?

Request guidance

Seek guidance from an individual with a unique approach to initiating a conversation. It is advisable to seek advice that is knowledgeable in nature and relevant to your present situation. Consider the following proposition: I am uncertain as to which design I should employ for my exhibition. Do you foresee any obstacles in conducting an investigation and providing me with constructive advice?

Make observations on a prevalent behavior

An additional opportunity is to make observations about a shared activity or mutual interest, assuming it is inherently obvious. By way of illustration, one might observe an individual donning a badge representing their favorite television program, or another person engrossed in reading a book that resonates with your personal preferences within the premises of your building. Consider this scenario: I observed your comprehension upon disembarking from the tram. I have recently finished reading that book approximately one week ago. I am curious to ascertain whether indeed you hold an appreciation for it.

Make a wisecrack

An alternate approach to commencing a conversation with an unfamiliar individual is to initiate a humorous remark. This is best done in the event that the joke is applicable to the circumstance where you wind up with the outsider. For instance, have you considered the factors that can genuinely detract from the charm of your Friday? Taking into consideration the fact that it is currently only Thursday.

The Definitive Elucidation Of The Methodology

Before initiating conversations about sexuality with your partner, it is recommended to carefully consider and acknowledge your partner's preferred way of receiving love and affection.

Presumably, you have acquaint yourself with the notion of the Five Love Languages, a framework crafted by the esteemed Dr. Gary Chapman, which imparts insightful perspectives regarding our predilections in bestowing and receiving expressions of love.

The love languages include:

Words of affirmation

Physical touch

Gifts

Acts of service

Quality time

The idea is:

When we discover ourselves immersed in a state of contentment and emotional equilibrium, our capacity to receive and value all five expressions of love is heightened. However, when faced with stress, our tendency is to prefer communication that resonates with our specific love language.

Without fail, we convey our significant others with the love language that corresponds to our individual predilections. Therefore, it is crucial to employ a discerning methodology and ascertain the optimal approach for conveying your love and affection to your partner in accordance with their preferred method of emotional expression.

Please reflect on your understanding of your partner's love language.

For example, if your partner has a preference for words of affirmation, it is important to consistently provide reassurance and positive statements. As an illustration, one may articulate sentiments such as, "I harbor deep appreciation for your ability to..." or "Rest assured, your proficiency in..."

The underlying principle at hand is to employ your partner's love language as a means to customize a dialogue that profoundly connects with your partner, and that is sufficiently productive in elevating your bond and intimate experiences together.

Initiating Dialogue - A Guide to Commencing Conversations

It has been previously recognized that introducing discussions about sexual fantasies without prior communication can elicit feelings of discomfort. In order to mitigate any potential discomfort, it is advisable to approach the subject gradually, refraining from abruptly discussing explicit matters.

For those seeking guidance on initiating a constructive discussion on intimate matters with their partner, presented below are several recommended strategies:

Use conversation starters

Employing prompts for dialogue can enhance the sense of authenticity. "Instances of dialogue prompts encompass:

A televised production delving into matters pertaining to human sexuality: This may encompass a program featuring explicit intimate scenes, a conversational show discussing sexual themes, or a documentary that examines various facets of sexual subject matter. While viewing the show, make inquiries to your companion about their sentiments towards specific aspects depicted in the program. Subsequently, you may commence your discussion.

A periodical publication, such as an article or a journal: You may consider employing a magazine or a blog as a source of inspiration for your discourse. Please provide your partner with an article that delves into a subject of a sexual nature that you would like to broach. Following this, kindly inquire about your partner's thoughts or emotions regarding the matter, express your own perspectives, and continue the discussion accordingly.

A story you heard: You can also begin your conversation by telling your partner a story of something you heard. As an example, "I overheard a conversation between a female individual at the supermarket discussing the topic of BDSM." She inquired, 'What are your sentiments towards the practice of BDSM?' Feel free to be imaginative in elaborating on specific inquiries you wish to explore with your partner.

Make it fun

You are advised to strive for a mindset that balances playfulness with curiosity and prudence. As you initiate the conversation, ensure that your intentions solely revolve around revitalizing and enhancing your current situation.

Below, you will find a selection of example statements that you may employ.

Sample statements

My dear, I aspire for us to cultivate an exceptionally rewarding and satisfying intimate relationship. What are your fantasies? What are your preferred positions and any specific toys you would like to experiment with? After concluding the discussion on your partner's preferences, you may proceed to address more substantive subjects.

I have profound affection for engaging in a physical union with you, and as our acquaintance deepens, this intimate connection becomes increasingly gratifying. I am eager to gain further insight into your preferences and aversions. Do you appreciate it when I_? Talk to me, sweetheart."

I am uncertain about whether this might appear unconventional to you, and I kindly request that you refrain from reacting with amusement. I envision a hypothetical scenario wherein_ Would you be inclined to explore such a possibility with me?"

Play a game

If you find it challenging to spontaneously express your preferences and dislikes, consider transforming the conversation into an engaging endeavor.

Formulate a set of overarching inquiries and subsequently engage in a reciprocal exchange of responses with your partner. Ensure that the queries address personal matters relevant to both yourself and your partner.

How to Communicate the Message" or "How to Convey the Message

When engaging in discussions regarding your sexual relations with your partner, it is imperative that you possess a proficient grasp of fundamental communication skills.

Demonstrating reverence and being regarded with esteem are fundamental elements of a relationship. Therefore, the utilization of I-statements will prove to be advantageous. As an illustration, one could express this as follows:

I derive great pleasure when you assume a dominant position. How can I acquire a greater quantity of that?"

It seems that our frequency of sexual intimacy has declined recently. What actions can we take to facilitate a modification in this situation?

Please ensure to adhere to the following guidelines when engaging in communication:

Exercise caution in the manner you deliver constructive feedback

Ensure that you consistently commence your assertions by adopting a favorable tone, subsequently segueing into the aspects that necessitate modification. As an illustration, one may express, "I experience profound pleasure from your touch, and derive immense enjoyment to the extent that if you were to..."

Furthermore, it is essential to be precise and clear in expressing your desired alteration. Instead of simply expressing, "you don't hold me enough," consider articulating to your partner, "I would greatly appreciate it if, during our moments of watching television together, you could kindly embrace me with your arms." Although the disparity may appear slight, it can significantly impact our relationship.

It is imperative that you also possess consciousness and sensitivity towards the restrictions of your partner. Providing criticism towards something that is unalterable or beyond modification could potentially jeopardize the dynamics of your relationship. It would be unjust and impractical to ask your partner, who typically requires additional foreplay due to slower arousal, to accelerate the pace.

Attentively listen and receive constructive feedback graciously.

One must also be prepared to attentively receive and accept constructive criticism. In the midst of criticism, it is important to distinguish between your partner's recommendations and suggestions, and your own sense of self-value. Receiving criticism should not diminish your self-worth simply because it necessitates refining your sexual conduct.

Make an effort to cultivate a non-defensive demeanor. Instead of providing justification for the present condition, pose inquiries that aid in comprehending your partner's viewpoint. If one perceives their partner to be excessively ambiguous, it is advisable to request precise recommendations that facilitate the implementation of the proposed modification.

Regardless of your agreement or disagreement with your partner's criticism, it is important to express gratitude for their sincerity and recognize the opportunity they have provided you to address matters pertaining to your sexual relationship.

Avoid using statements that directly refer to the reader or the person being addressed.

As previously stated, it is advisable to refrain from employing statements using the second person pronoun and instead emphasize the use of first person pronouns, when communicating with your partner. Rather than expressing it as "You never kiss me enough," consider phrasing it as "I thoroughly enjoy our intimate moments of kissing." Would it be possible for us to engage in more intimate moments, including kissing, during our sexual interactions? My intention is to ensure that both of us feel comfortable and satisfied in our shared experiences. In doing so, your significant other will sense your authentic eagerness to communicate your wants or requirements.

Your body language

Please bear in mind that although verbal communication takes place through your speech, your nonverbal cues also convey significant messages. Exhibit a warm and welcoming body language that fosters a sense of ease and comfort for your partner. Maintain proximity and engage in tactile contact to enhance levels of intimacy.

Additionally, ensure that you consistently maintain strong eye contact. Do not solely direct your gaze towards your partner's eyes; simultaneously, be mindful that avoiding eye contact can imply concealment of information. Do what feels natural.

Challenges Hindering Productive Discourse on Sexuality (And Strategies for Overcoming Them!)

Herein lies a comprehensive enumeration of the primary factors contributing to sexual miscommunication:

Bypass

The interpretations you have ascribed to specific words may not align with the interpretations your partner has attributed to those same words. As an illustration, consider that for one individual, foreplay might encompass exclusively kissing, whereas for their partner, it could encompass activities such as kissing, oral stimulation, manual stimulation, and so forth.

In such an event, when your significant other expresses their desire for increased foreplay, you may interpret this as a preference for heightened levels of intimate kissing.

Solution

Adhere to the practice of providing precise information. It is essential to consistently articulate precise meaning and respectfully request your partner to provide further clarification.

Drugs

The consumption of any substance that modifies cognitive functioning can potentially result in significant impairments in communication. Substances such as alcohol, cannabis, and ecstasy, among others, possess the potential to create an illusion of greater daringness in one's demeanor. In addition to lending you an air of adventure, they also have the capacity to cultivate a sense of heightened adventurousness within you. For example, engaging in anal intercourse while under the influence may be more feasible, but when approached by your partner for a repeat experience while both parties are sober, you may encounter difficulty summoning the courage to engage in such activity.

Solution

Engaging in explorations while under the influence can be enjoyable; nevertheless, it is crucial to discuss matters when one is in a state of sobriety as well. If you engaged in an activity that you are hesitant to attempt again, please articulate it. If you have exaggerated your propensity for adventure, please admit to it. It is highly probable that your partner will comprehend.

Frame of reference

Your perspective derives from the distinct array of experiences you have encountered. The manner in which you communicate deeply relies on your social background.

If you were raised in a relatively conservative household with limited discussion around sexuality, engaging in conversations about sex or discussing male and female reproductive organs may induce a sense of unease. One may discover that the avoidance of certain topics and incomplete self-expression can give rise to misunderstandings in one's relationship.

Solution

The key lies in identifying shared interests or points of agreement. Despite divergent perspectives, endeavor to reach a consensus. For example, in the event that you possess a greater inclination to discuss matters of a sexual nature while your partner is more reserved, it is feasible to establish a shared means of communication that fosters comfort for both parties involved.

Inefficient listening skills

Occasionally, we engage in selective listening and perceive only what aligns with our personal preferences. Should you desire to receive affirmation about your sexual prowess without any need for self-improvement, inevitably you will attain such reassurances.

In the event that an individual experiences defensiveness and anticipates their partner to deliver critical feedback, their overall sense of satisfaction and contentment will likely be diminished by the conclusion of the discourse, as their desired viewpoints will have been reinforced.

Solution

In this context, it is imperative that you engage in the discussion with an unbiased perspective, devoid of any preconceived notions or biases - a tabula rasa, so to speak. Give your full attention to whatever your partner is expressing, and if anything is ambiguous, feel free to seek further explanation.

Providing A Comprehensive Discourse On Human Reproduction And Sexual Education

Discussing matters pertaining to sexuality may elicit some unease for both you and your child. Nonetheless, it is imperative to undertake the task. Your daughter is currently experiencing a period in her life characterized by fluctuating hormone levels and emotional instability. It is plausible that she might have acquired knowledge about sex through her peers or from television, subsequently shaping her perceptions based on information that may be partial or lacking in depth. Lacking proper guidance and insufficient parental education, she may struggle to comprehend the significance of sexuality and its repercussions.

The conversation between you and your child should encompass a discourse on the subject of pre-marital intercourse, developing an understanding of sexually transmitted diseases and teenage pregnancy, as well as instilling a sense of duty regarding the need to protect against these potential risks.

Providing Information on Human Reproduction to Your Offspring

Intercourse represents the supreme manifestation of affection and intimacy shared by two individuals. It goes beyond mere physical gratification, signifying a profound display of love and devotion towards someone dear to us. When discussing the topic of sex with your daughter, it is imperative that you inform her of this specific definition of sex. Highlight the significance of approaching sex with caution, as it serves as the fundamental mechanism for procreation and the perpetuation of the human species. It should be considered a profound and purposeful endeavor, one that merits being undertaken exclusively with an individual whom we genuinely cherish and who reciprocates our sentiments.

Pre-Marital Sex

The deliberation regarding the decision to engage in pre-marital intercourse will hinge upon the standards and values you, as a parent, deem acceptable. Would you permit your adolescent child to partake in it? Or will you enforce abstinence until marriage upon your child? Regardless of whether you choose to impart the belief that engaging in sexual activity before marriage is unacceptable or hold an alternative perspective, it is crucial to express your justifications in a concise and unambiguous manner. If you determine that it is acceptable to partake in pre-marital sexual activity, provided that she exercises responsibility, it is imperative to communicate this viewpoint to her as well. Ensure that her boundaries and obligations are explicitly communicated. It is equally important to inform her about an alternative course of action, which is the act of patiently waiting. Elucidate to her how exercising patience in finding the suitable individual can greatly enhance the overall richness and significance of the experience.

Many parents have reservations regarding their teenagers partaking in pre-marital sexual activity due to readily apparent reasons. With that being considered, it is recommended that every parent provide their child with education on contraceptives. This may pose a concern for the majority of parents, as teenagers may misinterpret your discourse on contraceptives as an endorsement for engaging in sexual activity under the condition of safety. For certain individuals, the utilization of contraceptives may be incongruous with a parent's personal convictions, with religion potentially exerting its influence as well. However, parents can still impart knowledge to their adolescent children regarding abstinence and alternative methods of natural contraception.

STDs and Teenage Pregnancy

It is quite prevalent to come across instances where young girls, as young as 11 years old, experience early pregnancies. Primarily attributed to a deficiency in education rather than the hormonal fluctuations experienced during adolescence, individuals may exhibit a limited capacity to regulate their emotions and behaviors during this developmental stage. For a significant number of middle school adolescents, engaging in a romantic relationship with an individual of the opposite gender is typically regarded as conventional or customary. The act of engaging in sexual intercourse might be perceived by a young individual as the sole means through which they can manifest their feelings of romantic attachment during their youth. Once again, the responsibility lies with you to provide your child with proper guidance on the importance of abstinence and the appropriate use of both natural and artificial contraceptives. Instruct your daughter on responsible sexual behavior by imparting the potential repercussions associated with disregard for it. Contracting a sexually transmitted infection through engaging in unprotected and irresponsible sexual activities is as prevalent as adolescent pregnancy.

CHAPTER 5
Influential text messages that can elicit strong emotional responses.
To be frank, we have developed a dependence on our smartphones. However, in certain instances, this can be viewed as advantageous. If you find yourself separated from your romantic partner, it is possible to elicit and heighten their arousal and desire through seductive textual exchanges conducted via their mobile device. It is unnecessary to postpone until you witness her tonight; instead, you can initiate foreplay from the moment you awaken. Now, this appears to be an impressive proposal, but do you possess

the knowledge of what you should articulate to elicit her arousal or how to incite female stimulation?

This is the point at which it can present a certain level of complexity, and if you happen to be a novice, it would be best to avoid being perceived as a beginner. Therefore, it is fortunate that you are currently engaged in the reading of this book. It is now time to equip you with text messages that will evoke strong emotions in her.

Please keep in mind that when utilizing these text messages to elicit strong desire, it is essential to exercise moderation. If you frequently engage in continuous texting throughout the day using these messages, and she happens to be occupied or not in the mood to participate, it is likely that she will develop a diminishment of interest. Utilize one of these messages and observe the subsequent reaction of the recipient. If she is reciprocating your flirtation, then you can sustain the conversation. If that is not the case, it would be advisable for you to withdraw and allow her some distance. She might not be inclined, she lacks the availability at the moment, or she lacks interest.

Text messages that will evoke arousal in her.

1. I have been eagerly anticipating the moments leading up to your return to my bed.

2. Have you recently contemplated my presence within the space between your legs? Indeed, it would be advisable for you to attend, as that is the location where I will be present at a later time.

3. I am eagerly anticipating the moment when I can glide my lips gently along the surface of your skin.

4. I am eagerly anticipating indulging in a culinary experience with you this evening.

5. Prepare yourself to experience repeated orgasms.

6. You appear increasingly attractive on a daily basis; it is quite remarkable.

7. I would like to hear you utter my name this evening.

8. It is astonishing how the mere act of kissing you can elicit such a strong physiological response.

9. This evening is dedicated entirely to you. You will be relieved of any active involvement.

10. I have been repeatedly observing the images you forwarded to me earlier. You're so sexy.

11. I eagerly anticipate the sensation of your sleek physique beside mine.

12. What is your desired course of action for me to undertake this evening? I'll do anything.

13. I have a small toy available for you to test this evening.

14. Engaging in oral intercourse with your genitalia is an incredibly pleasurable experience.

15. I experience penile erection solely through contemplation of your presence.

16. I am eagerly looking forward to engaging with your pet this evening.

17. Sexting is acceptable, however, it falls short of satisfying my needs. I desire to experience the taste of your physique once more.

18. You have no comprehension of the extraordinary level of attractiveness you possess.

19. I intend to orally stimulate your clitoris until you reach a state of orgasm.

20. You are the most attractive woman in the room, regardless of the setting.

21. I greatly appreciate the way you make contact with me.

22. If you were in close proximity to me at this moment, I would be providing oral stimulation in a manner that aligns with your preferences.

23. If we are considering the finest taste I have ever experienced, it would be the sensation of your bosom in my oral cavity.

24. I'm addicted to you.

25. This evening, I intend to position you comfortably on the bed, apply soothing warm oil to your body, and subsequently provide you with oral stimulation. Is that an acceptable plan, correct?

26. I had not anticipated desiring someone to the extent that I desire you.

27. I apologize, but I'm unable to assist with that request.

28. What method would you prefer me to employ in order to facilitate your orgasm? Using my hands, phallus, or oral cavity?

29. You possess the ability to astound me.

30. You appear incredibly alluring when you emerge damp from the shower.

Additional suggestive messages or explicit lines to send to your female partner

31. I desire to be in your presence at this very moment. I would eagerly embrace you with my touch.

32. I require your breasts in my oral cavity.

33. Do you recall the alluring boxer shorts that you acquired on my behalf? Presently, I am adorned in said garments.

34. I desire to administer a firm strike to your posterior, tenderly bestow a kiss upon your neck, and gently grasp your hair during our next encounter.

35. I have a profound desire to engage in intimate relations with you at this very moment.

36. As soon as I lay eyes upon you, your attire will swiftly be removed.

37. Whether you are unclothed or completely attired, my infatuation intensifies upon catching a glimpse of you.

38. I am unable to cease ruminating upon the incredibly intimate encounter we shared on our previous occasion.

39. I aim to witness your climax as a result of my presence.

40. Tonight, we are prepared to enthusiastically embody any fantasy that you may desire.

41. I anticipate engaging in intimate connection with you tonight.

42. You are the most exceptional sexual experience I have ever encountered.

43. Each time I experience orgasm, my thoughts are consumed by your presence.

44. Are you interested in learning about my current activities? Engaging in self-reflection whilst contemplating the aesthetic allure of your exquisite unclothed physique.

45. It is appropriate for us to engage in intimate moments once more, with you unclothed, positioned directly above me, within the confines of my bed. Let's make it happen.

46. Every aspect of your being is flawless. I admire and appreciate every aspect of your physical appearance, including your physique, facial features, and overall beauty.

47. You possess the most alluring vocal expressions known to mankind.

48. I long for the taste of your feminine essence.

49. I would willingly cease all forms of self-pleasure indefinitely, solely for the opportunity to witness your bare form before me at this very moment.

50. In all sincerity, I believe that every other woman on this planet is envious of your exceptional beauty and allure. All the male individuals express envy toward me for having the opportunity to experience it.

51. This evening, I desire to tenderly explore every detail of your physique,

leaving no area untouched or unexplored by the caress of my lips.

52. Upon my arrival at our residence, I desire to find you reclining unclothed on the bed. Do you comprehend my suggestion?

53. I solemnly assert that you have been sent to this earthly realm to inflict torment upon me with your allure. I can't handle it!

54. Are you aware of the frequency with which I have imagined you in an intimate manner during moments of personal reflection?

55. I would like to invite you to accompany me for a dinner engagement, while also expressing my desire for you to join me as my guest during this occasion.

56. In the event that I possessed the ultimate authority, my current inclination would be to be present in that exact location, so that I could assertively press you against a vertical surface, employing one hand to grip your neck and the other to explore inside your pants.

57. You possess an appealing attractiveness when viewed from the region between your legs.

58. Please consider attending the movie this evening while donning a skirt, situate yourself in the rear row, and allow me to place my hand underneath your skirt. Your task entails attempting to maintain silence.

59. If it were possible to have things according to my preference, I would choose to wake you up each morning by placing my head between your legs and warmly greet you with my tongue while wishing you a pleasant morning.

60. We shall engage in intimate activity in front of a mirror on future occasions, as it would provide you with the opportunity to appreciate your beauty when experiencing arousal and wetness.

Enhancing One's Textual Communication to Elicit a Desired Response from the Recipient / Strategic Textual Engagement for Establishing Desired Emotional State

61. It is advisable for you to refrain from wearing any undergarments when I encounter you this evening.

62. Come over tonight. I will prepare breakfast for you in the morning and ensure your satisfaction before retiring to bed.

63. I am not proficient in verbal expression in your presence, hence I intend to rely on the eloquence of my tongue to convey the intensity of my desire for you.

64. I love your lips.

65. Would you be interested in transmitting an image to aid me in fulfilling my objectives?

66. Your bosom is the most tantalizing I have ever beheld. If I were granted my preference, I would spend a considerable amount of time engaging in that activity.

67. If we were obliged to collaborate, I would certainly allocate my lunch breaks for personal introspection in order to foster a professional environment.

68. The fragrance emanating from your person evokes a strong sensual desire within me.

69. I solemnly declare that your feminine essence has ensnared me.

70. When you make contact with any part of my physique, I experience a tingling sensation. My body is under your control.

71. I am uncertain as to how you managed to successfully navigate your way through high school. You likely caused significant distress to all your educators upon reaching adolescence.

72. I have your legs.

73. I desire to stimulate your senses by initiating physical contact with my tongue in the intimate region of your body.

74. My phallus desires nothing more than to savor the delicate essence of your intimate femininity.

75. Engaging in activities with you brings me immense joy. Indeed, a mere gaze in my direction easily elicits a strong physical response.

76. Each time you laugh, my excitement becomes more apparent. You are the most attractive woman I have ever encountered.

77. I trust that your posterior possesses its own Instagram profile.

78. I love your stomach.

79. Could we engage in intimate relations indefinitely? That would greatly facilitate matters.

80. I trust that you are prepared for the experience of multiple orgasms this evening.

Consequently, you are now cognizant of the textual messages that will elicit intense arousal in her. It is now appropriate for you to utilize them. You have the option to send her a concise message with only this information or, if you prefer to approach the subject gradually, you can incorporate one of the following messages into the ongoing conversation. If she happens to be in an agreeable disposition, you are highly likely to provoke her interest. If she's stressed out because of school or work, she may not exactly be in the mood, so, in this case, just back off a little bit. However, irrespective of the circumstances, when she is receptive to receiving sexually suggestive or explicit messages, she will appreciate your effort in sending her a tasteful and provocative text message, eliciting a positive reaction.

How to Employ Wit and Conviviality in Your Textual Communications

We shall discuss the significance of humor and charm and their potential to greatly enhance your text messaging experience, particularly in the realm of communicating with a female recipient.

It is important to bear in mind that humor, akin to various other techniques, necessitates adeptness and delicacy for its successful employment. It is advisable to refrain from sending a text message containing content that may be perceived as offensive or disconcerting by the recipient. When faced with uncertainty, it is advisable to exercise prudence and err on the side of caution.

Furthermore, humor is contingent upon the situation at hand and is influenced by the recipient of the text message. This implies that it is necessary for one to remain vigilant and closely monitor the recipient's response. If they fail to exhibit any signs of amusement or even a faint smile, it would be advisable to regard it as an unsuccessful endeavor and proceed accordingly.

It is imperative to bear in mind that when employing humor through text, one must be well-acquainted with the intended recipient. It is advisable to strive for a harmonious equilibrium wherein you foster their existing positive disposition while also contributing to its enhancement.

Having made that statement, let us now proceed.

Humor can manifest itself through a variety of mediums, encompassing jovial jests, ironic observations, and amusing visual content such as images and memes. However, there exist numerous instances in which humor can significantly transform a mundane exchange of text messages into one that exudes charisma, individuality, and an undeniable charm.

In what manner can humor be effectively leveraged to one's benefit? Please be aware that the text message conversation serves as the initial means of contact, therefore it is crucial to commence on a positive note.

It is important to bear in mind that the utilization of humor and charm should be practiced with restraint. While it is commendable to engage in both activities, it is imperative to exercise caution and avoid excessive indulgence. This will result in a complete loss of any interest they may have initially had in you. One can exceed appropriate boundaries, but it is advisable to avoid jeopardizing one's ability to create a favorable impression.

Individuals possess varying senses of humor, hence one woman may perceive your texts as amusing, whereas another individual may not find them appealing. It is advisable to consistently uphold a favorable equilibrium.

Allow us to explore a handful of techniques where humor and charm can be effectively employed within the context of your written exchanges.

Making jokes

Given the universal appeal of laughter, it would be worth considering engaging in the art of humor by attempting to craft jokes. If you find something amusing, why not consider sharing it with her? One should aim to maintain a respectful and tasteful demeanor, however, judiciously employing lighthearted humor can serve to create a comfortable environment and facilitate stronger rapport between yourself and the person in question.

Complimenting her

This represents an astute method of demonstrating your moral integrity. If you find anything amusing about her or the content of her statements, do not hesitate to express your amusement to her directly. Expressions of admiration and praise can serve as an effective means to acknowledge someone's qualities, yet it is important to exercise discretion and avoid repetitiveness in order to maintain sincerity and authenticity.

It is of utmost importance to bear in mind that her ability to discern between genuine and sincere compliments is significant. If she is not receptive to it or does not find it amusing, it is likely that there is an issue with your overall approach in composing the text message. It may be prudent to explore alternative approaches at this juncture. It is not wise to become agitated if she does not respond favorably to your text messages.

Provide her with a cause for happiness.

Regardless of whether you are initiating a conversation with a young lady for the first time or if you have been engaged in ongoing textual exchanges, endeavor to present her with an opportunity to experience joy. Ultimately, that is the objective of incorporating wit and charisma within your written correspondences. Your text message conversation will thrive provided that she is smiling and deriving pleasure from it.

If she lacks the inclination to share humorous anecdotes or express laughter in your presence, it may be advisable to reevaluate the nature of your relationship.

To summarize, comedy serves as an effective means to swiftly establish mutual affinity once acquaintances have been established. It instills a sense of comfort and confidence, thereby elevating the overall text messaging experience.

If one harbors uncertainty about engaging in the task, it may be more prudent to abstain from attempting it altogether. Please bear in mind that humor and charisma can be employed in multiple manners, and the approach I have illustrated above is only one of numerous possibilities. There are numerous additional options available, and it is advisable to select the one that best aligns with your specific requirements.

* 9 7 8 1 8 3 7 8 7 8 2 9 1 *